Less Than Perfect Is Perfect

Less Than Perfect Is Perfect

LENSEY ACKERMAN

Edited by Andrew Dawson

Cover illustration: Olena Veres / Shutterstock

979-8-9921660-0-2 (paperback)

979-8-9921660-1-9 (ebook)

For my beautiful daughter, Maggey

*And for anyone who has struggled or is struggling
with perfectionism and/or body image issues.*

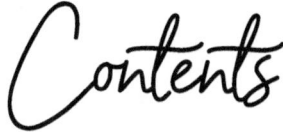

Contents

CHAPTER ONE

The Beginning

WHAT IS THE definition of perfection? Perfection is defined as the condition or quality of being free or as free as possible, from all flaws or defects. Now, this may not be of any significance to many people. But for me, I lived and breathed by this definition. It took me close to three decades to realize that this word cannot be used to define humanity, no matter how much we may strive for it. No human being can obtain true perfection, as every person has their own unique flaws. There is no such thing as a perfect human.

Everyone on this earth is different and unique, and no two individuals are the same. Can you imagine how boring and strange life would be if we were all alike? There are no specific characteristics or traits that qualify someone as perfect. Every man and woman has their own opinion of which qualities are the most desired and flawless. However, these opinions do not define what is perfect.

When I was born in the mid-eighties, I surely came into this world with the "perfectionist gene." From what I have been told and gathered on my own, I inherited this gene from my mother's side of the family. Apparently, my maternal grandfather, whom I never met, was very neat and orderly. He passed away when I was just a baby. Growing up, I remember our house was always spotless, and everything in our kitchen pantry was categorized and stored in labeled Tupperware containers. My mom worked very hard to keep our house of five neat and clean.

It wasn't until I was about seven or eight years old that it became obvious to me that I had some obsessive-compulsive disorder (OCD) tendencies. In other words, I was an extraordinary "neat freak." Every object on my dresser was in its precise spot and at the exact angle I wanted. Whenever I had a friend over to play, things would get moved out of place. Once I was alone again, I would immediately have to "fix" and reposition everything back to the way I had it. I must have spent so much time and energy on perfecting my room and my belongings.

I made my bed every single day, and it was always made according to my own personal standards. My twin brother never understood it. In fact, he loved to tease me and come jump on my bed and mess it all up, knowing how much it would bother me. It was so cruel, but we were just kids, and he was just being a typical brother. After this happened, I would immediately kick him out of my room and lock my door so that I could be alone and make my bed nice and neat again.

OCD, like many other disorders, is unique to every diagnosed individual. Signs and symptoms vary, and what may be true for one person may not be true for another. However, uncontrollable, recurring thoughts and/or behaviors are the common denominator among those with this disorder. During my childhood, my urge to reposition things repeatedly until it was "just right" was a true sign of my compulsive tendencies, a symptom of OCD.

It was difficult to be like this when my brother and sister seemed so "normal." I even had moments where I really disliked myself for being this way, and

I would find myself breaking down and crying after episodes of ordering and arranging. It was exhausting. This is not how I wanted to spend my time. It turns out that OCD is commonly downplayed and is actually listed as one of the top ten most debilitating psychiatric disorders (Cross Border Books, 2022).

I realize now how lucky I was that my only real "issue" during childhood was being overly and compulsively neat. I was physically healthy, and I had loving parents who cared so much for me and my siblings. I had a big sister who I looked up to, and a twin brother who I got to share every milestone with. We created so many wonderful family memories from holidays and road trips.

I was devoted to my schoolwork and getting good grades, and I worked hard to become a great tennis player. We had a tennis court in our backyard, so my dad spent many hours out there coaching us. There were days when he worked long hours, yet he would come home and go right out on the court to give us a lesson. Growing up in South Florida, we were also fortunate to have a boat, and we did a lot of tubing, snorkeling, and skiing. I was very blessed to have had such an amazing childhood.

Despite being an athlete and spending a lot of time playing with my twin brother and other neighborhood kids, I was still very much a girly girl. I loved Barbies and everything pink. I also loved to dress up and pretend I was a super model. My mom signed me up for a couple of child modeling gigs for department stores, but nothing serious. For as long as I can remember, I have dreamed of becoming a professional model one day. However, it didn't seem realistic to either me or my family. So, instead, I strived to become a great tennis player.

As I said, we had a tennis court in our backyard, so we were able to practice every day. It was so convenient and beneficial. Florida has always been known for training top players, so it was very competitive. I even grew up playing at some of the same tennis clubs where the Williams sisters played. I lived a very normal childhood, despite the many hours spent practicing tennis and the many weekends away from home playing in tournaments.

I didn't want tennis to be my entire life, which is usually what it takes to become a star. My goal was to be good enough to play for a Division I college team one day, and hopefully receive some scholarship money to do so. I still made time to socialize and play with friends, and I was very diligent with my schoolwork. Getting good grades always came first.

One thing is for sure, I always wanted to get better at everything I did. I never wanted to settle for mediocre. I was quite hard on myself at times. I would put myself under so much pressure to be better or accomplish more. It was never enough for me. That seemed to work both *for* me and *against* me. It just goes to show that I really was a perfectionist.

CHAPTER TWO

The Big Change

WHEN IT COMES to my upbringing, you could say that it was very Christian. My family was devoted to the church and attended every Sunday. My siblings and I enjoyed going to Sunday school. My grandparents, aunts, uncles, and cousins all went to the same church. My maternal grandmother was a very proper lady. She grew up in the Methodist church and was a very religious Christian. She didn't drink, and she never said a swear word. She also never went out in public without her make-up on, hair done, and being dressed to impress. If she could only see me now, going out to run errands in yoga pants, sneakers, and a baseball cap.

As you can imagine, my sister and I were both very innocent growing up. We had strict curfews and were not allowed to date until we were sixteen years old. When our friends got to stay out late at parties, we had to be home by midnight. In fact, we had very strong morals instilled in us that included avoiding sex until marriage. Growing up as a millennial, this was a very alien concept to most of my generation. Most of my friends were losing their virginity in high school. I tended to feel a little out of place and even envious of others because of this. However, I prided myself on the idea of "saving" myself for the one I loved and planned to marry, the one who was deserving of the one thing that no other guy would get to share with me. This was a lot more difficult for me during my college years, which I will get into more later.

One of the hardest times in my life was moving to Connecticut in the middle of my high school years. My dad was being transferred for work, so we had no choice but to leave Florida the summer before my junior year of high school. I was devastated. I was leaving the only town I knew and all the friends I grew up with or had become close to in the previous two years. I loved my high school. I was on the tennis team, and I had a huge group of friends. I truly felt loved and popular. I was at the top of my class, and I was planning to join the student government. I had so many opportunities to date, but I loved having guy friends and not being tied down with someone.

I will never forget the day we were officially leaving for Connecticut, when we were at the airport getting ready to board our flight. We were greeted by so many of our friends, about two dozen, who came to send us off. That is how loved my twin brother and I were. It was so special, yet extremely emotional. It was so hard to say goodbye and head into the unknown.

Being uprooted to a foreign state and town at such a vital age was very scary and surreal for me. I am so glad I had my twin brother by my side. We had to adjust to cold weather, a new high school, and we had to start from scratch making friends. We didn't know anybody. Meanwhile, we were only two years away from college, which meant we also had to start focusing on our post-graduation plans.

Of course, I joined the tennis team at the new high school, and eventually I made some close friends. However, it just wasn't the same. My heart was still in Florida where all my friends were, along with the high school I knew and loved. I never felt like I truly belonged to this school and town that I was thrown into. It was so different from what I was used to, and it was hard no longer being one of the popular students. I felt like an alien in a small, foreign town.

Despite the homesickness, I was able to get through those final two years of high school by focusing on my grades and tennis, and knowing that I would soon be leaving for college. It also helped that my brother and I made many trips back to Florida to visit our friends and go to their homecomings and proms, as if we had never left that high school. It was hard to understand at the time, but I realize now that I was very blessed to have friends in both places. In fact, it was at the school in Connecticut where I met a girl who is still my best friend to this very day.

I graduated high school with honors, and I was excited to begin the next chapter in my life. I received several offers for tennis scholarships from different colleges. It was an extremely hard decision, but I did not want to be too far away from home. I decided to go to the University of New Hampshire on a tennis scholarship. It was about a three-hour drive from our home in Connecticut, which I felt was a perfect distance.

There was a train station right on campus, which made it easy for my parents to visit and vice versa.

My college years were some of the best of my life, despite all that I went through during that time. My parents ended up getting a divorce, which was really for the best in the end. I am glad that I was old enough at that point to realize it, and I knew that it was necessary for the health of my parents and our family. It was still very difficult though, and it affected me more than I realized at the time. I was experiencing a lot of anxiety, and I didn't know how to manage it. I decided to start seeing a therapist on campus. I was exhibiting this compulsive behavior which, according to the therapist, was evidently a type of subconscious coping mechanism. It wasn't like the OCD tendencies I had growing up. This time it involved my body and physical appearance.

I am so thankful that I had the tennis team and sorority to help keep me busy and distracted. Between my studies, the demands of college tennis and, eventually, commitment to a sorority, I had very little time to focus on anything else. It was in the second semester of my sophomore year of college that I made the decision to join a sorority. I knew it would be a lot to balance with everything else. However, I always believed in the importance of "sisterhood" and healthy socialization. Even though I had my teammates and some other friends, I felt like I needed more. Joining Kappa Delta was one of the best decisions I ever made. I felt I belonged as soon as I joined, thanks to the love and support I received from the other girls, my "sisters." There was an instant connection.

A lot of people have a misconception that joining a fraternity/sorority is just about partying, and that you are "paying for your friends." While there is a lot of opportunity for partying in college Greek life, that is really the case for any college student whether part of an organization or not. My sorority experience was so much more than I even imagined it would be. I gained a huge support system, developed life-long friendships with many amazing and talented young women, and created some of the best memories of my life.

I had gained a lot of self-confidence during this time of my life. I owe so much of that to my sorority sisters, who always made me feel special and loved. It was so nice to be part of a group of young women who liked to build each other up. And we had so much fun! When I look back at pictures, I admire just how content

I was during those last couple of years in college. I was an athlete, so I was muscular. But, I was also skinny. I was above average in height and had long blonde hair. My sorority sisters nicknamed me "Barbie." I wore a size four in women's clothing and that was the largest size I had ever worn, both before and after college. I ate and drank a lot, like most college students do, but I stayed active. At that time, I was happy with myself.

When it came to determining my career plans, I was not one of the lucky ones who knew exactly what they wanted to do for a living. I initially started out with my college major listed as "undecided." I enjoyed biology and debated doing the pre-med program, but I was too afraid of failure and not being able to meet the demands. I ended up settling for a business degree in marketing.

The reason for feeling like I settled with my degree choice is that deep down I knew I wanted to be in healthcare. I loved learning about human anatomy, and anything related to health and nutrition. However, I did not believe I could satisfy the lofty standards necessary for a pre-med degree, in addition to my commitment to the tennis team and my scholarship. I guess you could say this was a true sign of my fear of failure and lack of self-confidence. I even considered becoming a nurse, but after witnessing my mother's nursing career, and all the "dirty work" it entailed, I just wasn't sure if that was for me. Truthfully, I wish I had believed in myself more. I was smart enough. I worked hard enough. I probably could have made it work if I had been more confident. I should have tried. Trying and failing is better than not trying at all.

CHAPTER THREE

Reality

AFTER I GRADUATED college, I decided to pursue a career in medical sales. Of course, in the medical device and pharmaceutical world, you need strong sales experience to land a good job with a reputable company. So, after graduation and having the opportunity to spend three months in Nantucket as a tennis professional (the best summer of my life), I took a job in outside sales for an office equipment company. I needed to put some quality experience on my resume. This was a tough job and required a significant amount of driving and "cold calling." The basic pay wasn't great, so there was a lot of pressure to earn commission.

During this time, I was living at home with my dad and stepmom in Connecticut. Most of my friends lived far away so I didn't have a whole lot going on outside of work. There really wasn't much to do in the small town where we lived, and the winters were so long. In fact, this is when I started to spend most of my free time exercising. I was playing tennis indoors, and I also joined a nearby gym. It was at this point that I started to become very focused on my body. I didn't like how muscular I was from being a college athlete and the intense weightlifting. I also felt like I didn't recognize myself in pictures because I weighed more than I ever did prior to college. I wanted to be skinny and lean. I even purchased and downloaded an entire book about "how to get six-pack abs." When I didn't feel like driving to the gym, I was able to work out in our basement, part of which had been converted to an exercise room. I became obsessed with this desire to look and feel like a model.

I decided to take it upon myself to invest in modeling school at John Casablanca's modeling agency, which was near where we lived. As I have said, I always wanted to be a model when I young, but I knew it was a "pipe dream." I saw this as more of a side-hustle and hobby. I really enjoyed it and learned a lot about the modeling industry. There are so many different components. I loved learning the correct ways to walk the runway. Walking the runway is so exhilarating! After completing the required courses and becoming an official "model" for the agency, there were many opportunities for small modeling gigs. The only problem was I was working full-time as a sales rep, so I only had the weekends available. Most of the modeling jobs were on specific days and scheduled at random times. I just didn't know how to make it work, as I still had to earn money and make a living. I couldn't rely on just those short-term modeling opportunities to support myself.

As much as I did not want to leave this area, due to being so close to the big modeling opportunities in New York City, I ended up making the decision to move back to my hometown in Florida. It was where my heart was. I was fortunate that I was able to transfer within my company, and my sister was kind enough to let me live with her in her condo for a while. I happened to be in a serious relationship at the time with a guy who also lived there, so we wouldn't have to struggle with the "long distance" aspect of our relationship anymore. This was just another benefit of moving back.

Once I got settled in Florida, I decided to search for the closest modeling agency. I needed to do a photo shoot and update my portfolio so that I could continue to pursue modeling. However, I came across the same difficulty as I had up north. I was still working full-time, and the good modeling opportunities were in Miami, which was a long drive from where I lived. I was in my early twenties and at a point in my life when I wasn't completely sure what I wanted to do or how to do it. I didn't have anyone encouraging or supporting me to pursue my dream of modeling. I ended up giving up on this altogether because I didn't believe I could do it. I had a muscular build from being an athlete, and I was only five feet, seven inches tall. Most successful models at the time were super tall and skinny, with no curves. It felt like I was being unrealistic to think I could have a successful career in that industry. Even if I was being naïve, I do wish that I had pursued it for longer because I did really enjoy it as a hobby.

CHAPTER FOUR

Love Wasn't Enough

I WAS SO miserable with my sales job, especially after transferring to Florida. The excessive amount of driving was beginning to take a toll on me. I knew it was time for a change, especially since I was not planning on having a life-long career in that industry. I had been with this company for two years, and it was strictly to gain the experience that I needed for medical device or pharmaceutical sales. I was not passionate about the products, and I did not like the amount of driving and cold calling that was involved with this particular job.

It wasn't easy depending on my sister for a place to live. I had hoped that one day my boyfriend and I would eventually get a place together. However, that dream soon faded. He was not motivated and decided to drop out of the local community college where he was taking classes to earn a bachelor's degree. He was just working part-time jobs and could barely afford to pay his own rent. This started to have an effect on me more than I was able to, or wanted to, acknowledge at the time. When it comes to matters of the heart, it can be easy to look the other way.

I finally made the decision to quit my job, with the complete support of my sister and family. They hated seeing how miserable I was. As I contemplated my next career move, I took a part-time job in a doctor's office, as an office assistant. I also worked as a tennis instructor and ran clinics at the local tennis club. I seriously contemplated going back to school for a graduate degree, but I was hesitant to start taking classes without knowing exactly what I was going to do. I did not like the idea of taking out loans to pay for everything.

During this time, while trying to figure out my own path, I was also trying to understand my boyfriend's goals and what his plans were for the future. He could barely afford to feed himself, let alone take me on a date of any kind. Even then, I still struggled to see how he was negatively influencing me and slowly bringing me down with him (unintentionally, of course). I found myself becoming more and more focused on my eating and exercise habits to cope with the stress and uncertainty in my life. I also felt as though I needed to compete with how skinny he was getting. He had stopped working out and wasn't eating much. I was very insecure about having a boyfriend who was skinnier than me. Unfortunately, this became the start of a real low point in my life. I felt like someone was slowly draining my motivation and confidence.

After my boyfriend ended up moving to North Carolina to live with his parents, I knew that signified the beginning of the end of any long-term plans I had hoped to make with him. So, here I was with no full-time job, no boyfriend, no place of my own, with crushed dreams and a broken heart. To help myself feel as though I still had some semblance of control in my life, I continued to restrict my eating and calorie intake and work out excessively at the gym. Not only was my body not getting enough energy to keep up with the calories I was burning, but I was also becoming a hermit. My usual "social butterfly" self was declining invitations to go out with friends to avoid the temptations and calorie consumption of eating and drinking. I wouldn't let myself go have a bagel with my sister on a Sunday morning or enjoy more than a single slice of pizza on a Friday night. I spent a lot of time in my room alone. My sister didn't know how to help me. I know it was very difficult for her to witness this.

I was still communicating with my "boyfriend" long distance because I truly missed him and, deep down, I still had a glimmer of hope for us. My dad, who was still living in Connecticut, reached out to me a lot via e-mail. I have always been very close to my dad and valued his input and advice about anything and everything. His opinion always mattered. One day, he brought to my attention in an e-mail that there was no future for me with this guy. This wasn't just any guy, though. He was the one on whom I had the biggest crush and admired since high school. He was the one I had daydreamed about being with but didn't think it would ever happen.

It was so hard for me to digest and accept this input from my dad, like a knife to my heart. However,

I knew he was right. I had been on a downward spiral ever since I moved back to Florida and was with him. I realized that I did not want to go backwards anymore. It felt like I had been wasting precious time, and I knew that I wanted much more for myself. I did not recognize this person I had become, and it would only get worse before it got better.

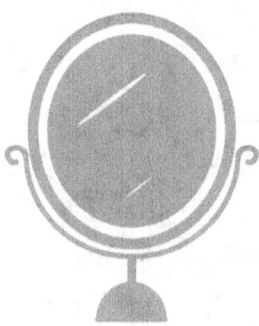

CHAPTER FIVE

The Disorder

BREAKING UP WITH my first love, who I thought could be the one, was one of the hardest things I had ever done. I didn't even have the courage to do it over the phone, which is awful. It was too difficult for me. I still loved him, and I never wanted things to turn out this way. But he gave me no choice. I needed to move forward with my life and take care of myself. In an e-mail, I told my boyfriend that I needed a break to focus on myself and get my life together. However, it hurt him knowing that my family had lost hope in him, and he could sense that I too had become doubtful. His own mother even told him that he needed to let me go because I deserved better. At this point he had pretty much given up on us, and even himself it seemed, so there was no longer a future for "us." It was very disappointing that he didn't even try to fight for that future. This is when I learned one of life's hard lessons: that love is not always enough, and you cannot change a person, especially if they don't want to change.

As part of the healing process and getting back on the right path, which included taking care of myself, I made the difficult decision to see a therapist. I needed someone who I could talk to without judgement, and who would listen to me and help me navigate my feelings and behaviors. It was time to regain my mental and physical health, while healing from a broken heart. It was hard to admit that I needed help. I have always been the type of person who will try to figure things out on my own. I do not like depending on others or asking for help. At that point in time, I still didn't fully recognize that I had a serious illness. It turns out that not only was I struggling with body image issues, or body dysmorphia, but I was also battling an eating disorder commonly known as anorexia.

It had gotten bad. No matter how much weight I lost, or how skinny I was, it was not enough for me. The sad thing is, when I looked in the mirror, I didn't see what others saw. I didn't see a girl, who was once a college athlete, withering away and losing her muscle mass because her body was starving. In fact, I liked the way I looked. I was fully in the grip of the disease.

I will never forget the doctor's appointment that changed my life. Even though I was seeing a therapist and getting help, I still wasn't totally convinced that I was harming my body. Like most mental illnesses, accepting that one has an issue is usually the biggest hurdle. Clearly, the doctor could see that I was underweight. However, what she really needed to know was what repercussions it was having on the inside of my body. I can tell you that never once had it occurred to me that I was putting my body and my health in danger. And even if I had realized it, I am not sure it would have made a difference. An eating disorder is a serious mental illness, a battle of the mind. It is a very difficult disease to overcome. In my mind, I was just controlling my weight and appearance. It didn't occur to me that I was starving my body and organs in the process.

My family and friends were very worried about me, and rightfully so. I couldn't see what they were seeing. I thought I looked great, and I was in control of my body. But they saw me as very frail and too skinny. My grandfather thought I was slowly killing myself. I had no body fat, and I was even beginning to lose my muscle as well. People kept trying to force food on me that I did not want to eat. I wouldn't eat a single piece of chocolate for fear of what it would do to me. Sometimes, I would feel pressured to accept a piece of cake or something I did not want (because it was "fattening") just so that the person would not think I had a problem. Little did they know that I would secretly throw it away later, pretending that I had eaten it. Hello, eating disorder.

I had gone more than two years without having a menstrual cycle. I had no idea at the time that there was a name for this condition: functional hypothalamic amenorrhea (FHA). Because my body did not have enough fat, it was being deprived of one of its most vital female functions. When it comes to reproduction, body fat plays a significant role. My extremely low body mass index (BMI) was preventing my body from producing enough estrogen, resulting in my inability to have a menstrual cycle for so long. If I was not having a routine monthly cycle then I was not releasing any eggs from my ovaries, due to the lack of hormones. When the reproductive hormone, estrogen, isn't stimulated, you're at a much higher risk of osteoporosis in addition to being unable to bear children.

After the tests and bloodwork results came back from the doctor's office, I was faced with a harsh reality. At the tender age of twenty-three, I was already developing osteopenia in my right hip. My bones, as well as other vital organs in my body, were not getting the nutrients they needed to be healthy and function properly. This really scared me because my grandmother had osteoporosis, and I knew it was too soon for me to be experiencing bone loss.

It was during this time that I was also informed by my doctor that I may never be able to fulfill my dream of having my own children one day. This news was absolutely devastating. I had always dreamed of becoming a mother. I even had a name already picked out for the baby girl I hoped to have one day. However, I was doing some serious damage to my ovaries. Despite being unintentional, I couldn't believe that I had done this to myself. This was the real turning point for me.

It was time to take the necessary steps, with the help of my therapist and family, to get my health back on track. I needed to start "reprogramming" my brain to no longer see food as an enemy but as the source of energy and life for my body and organs. Yes, this is a lot easier said than done. Habits are not easy to break. Exercise is in my DNA, and it's a vital part of living a healthy life, so I was not going to quit that. However, cutting back on the frequency and duration of the workouts, as well as adequately replenishing my body afterwards, was crucial for my health.

This was tough for me. For quite some time, this was the one area in my life where I truly felt like I had control. When other things in my life were not going as planned, I was able to put my focus on my physical appearance I decided how much food I ate and how often I exercised. This sense of control allowed me to feel better about myself and how my body looked. However, it became clear to me that this was really harming my body more than it was helping. I had no intentions of risking my health, or even my life, so I knew it was time to start changing my habits. It was obvious that this was going to take time and not something I was going to accomplish overnight.

CHAPTER SIX

Enterprise

A SIGNIFICANT FACTOR in getting myself healthy again was determining the next step in my career path and getting a new full-time job. I needed to get a sense of control and stability back in my life so that I would not feel so stressed and "lost." A girlfriend of mine convinced me to apply for a job with Enterprise, the car rental company where she worked. Despite my hesitation and lack of desire to work there, I decided to give it a try and joined their management trainee program. Not in a million years would I have foreseen myself working in the rental car industry. It did not excite me by any means, but I had to remind myself that this was just a stepping-stone to where I was destined to be.

There was nothing easy or glamorous about working for Enterprise. In fact, it involved long days and a significant amount of manual labor. However, this job enabled me to share an apartment with a roommate, so I no longer needed to rely on my sister for support. I was still young, in my mid-twenties, and I was still discovering who I was and the woman I wanted to become. Getting an apartment with my girlfriend was an exciting step towards becoming a better me.

The management training program at Enterprise attracted many other young adults like me. They were fresh out of school, motivated, and wanted to build a career by working towards a management position within the company. This required a significant amount of "blood, sweat, and tears," as they say. I worked ten to twelve-hour days, and sometimes seven days straight before having a day off. A typical day entailed answering the phone, booking reservations, greeting customers when they walked in, renting them a car, selling them the insurance coverage, and providing the best customer service possible. However, every day was different, and it was rarely easy.

There were some days when we wouldn't have a single car available to rent, or we didn't have enough cars to meet the number of reservations we had. Too often, our employee who cleaned the cars was absent, so we had to clean them ourselves (inside and out). People love to trash rental cars, let me tell you. I remember so many times that I would be outside vacuuming and washing a car at 7:30 a.m., in my nice, professional work clothes. And forget about wearing high heels because that was impossible with this job. Also, there were so many irrational customers and/or those who did not qualify to rent a car. Sounds fun, doesn't it? Those long, labor-intensive days made it hard for me to find time or energy for anything else. But some evenings I still managed to make it to the gym right after work.

I enjoyed going to the gym to work out and feel better about myself, but it also became more of a healthy way to relieve stress. It allowed me to escape the pressures and demands of the day. I was no longer doing it in excess either, now that I was working long days. I would put my headphones on, listen to music, and just focus on my workout. But I wouldn't overdo it or stay for longer than an hour.

When it came to my health, I was making progress. At this point, I was still seeing a therapist regularly, although not as frequently as before. I was no longer counting my calories, or at least not as much as before, and I usually packed myself a healthy lunch and snacks. Sometimes I would even splurge and order take-out food with co-workers. I was very diligent about taking a daily multivitamin and a calcium chew to help repair my bones. Also, I was making new friends at Enterprise, and we enjoyed getting together outside of work. This was a good turning point for me.

When my menstrual cycle started again, after two years without one, I felt immediate relief and knew that my body was getting healthy. I felt hopeful that I could still have kids one day, but I knew there was the possibility that I had done some permanent damage to my reproductive system. I learned so much from this difficult experience. As much as I had always idolized super skinny and lean women, I had never understood how important it is for a female to have a certain amount of body fat. In fact, it is necessary for a woman's health and well-being, and perhaps even the survival of humanity.

Seeing a therapist and having someone to talk to, without any judgement, is by far the healthiest decision I have ever made. It's a form of self-care that should really be encouraged and considered by everyone. One should never be ashamed of seeking advice from a professional therapist. It truly helps, and, in my opinion, I don't think there is a single human out there who would not benefit from it.

It is undeniable that my early to mid-twenties were a tough period for me. I cried many tears during the five years that I was working for Enterprise. This sounds awful, I know. But I learned a lot about myself and my capabilities during this stage of my life. The days were long and rigorous, and I had to work crazy hours sometimes sometimes, with shifts starting as early as 4 am and others finishing as late as 1 am. I always got through it though and knew that it was temporary.

I have always been very sensitive, but this job helped me gain a "thick skin" when it came to dealing with customers and people in general. I learned to not take things personally and to accept that some people are just mean and miserable. I also came to understand that I am not the kind of person who gives up. I keep working towards my goal, no matter what. And if, and when, I fall, I will get back up.

My goal while working at Enterprise was to prove to myself and to others that I could become a branch manager. It may have been a position predominately filled by men, but I knew I could do it and other females were doing it as well. You had to compete against others in an interview to get promoted. This came easier to some than others. A lot of it also had to do with who you knew within the company.

I witnessed many employees, including some of my close friends, who could not stick it out. They couldn't handle the demands of the job or the environment. Most of them either quit or stopped trying until they were let go. After a few promotions and almost four years with the company, I finally reached my goal of becoming a branch manager. My hard work and perseverance had paid off, and I was officially chosen to oversee my own branch and lead several employees.

Having a management career at Enterprise was not my life-long dream, nor was it part of a long-term plan. It was a journey with an inevitable ending. However, despite everything, there was a lot of good that came from my experience with Enterprise. Not only did I learn more about myself and what I was capable of, but I made so many genuine friends, including four girls who are still my coach friends to this very day. Since most of us were young and single at the time, we enjoyed many fun nights together at the bars and dance clubs. We all worked so hard, so we deserved to occasionally unwind and have some fun. I even discreetly dated a couple of my male co-workers. During my time working there, I was able to get my life back on track and become a healthy version of myself again.

I especially do not regret the time spent working at Enterprise because it was there where I ended up meeting the man who would one day become my husband. I was working for a satellite office within a Mercedes dealership, and I remember running into this tall, handsome guy with blonde, spikey hair who worked for Mercedes. I did not think anything of it at first, mostly because I was not looking to date anyone at the time. I could also tell that there was an age gap.

CHAPTER SEVEN

Mr. Right

AS YOUNG GIRLS, we tend to create this image in our minds of exactly what our ideal partner, the "man of our dreams," is going to be like. This guy at work was different from the portrayal I had envisioned in my mind. He was older than me and already had a daughter from a previous relationship (which I had found out from a colleague). However, I became friends with a couple of his co-workers who happened to be close friends of his. I met up with them one evening as they were out celebrating his birthday. To cut a long story short, we ended up at a club later that night and I asked him to dance with me. And so, our relationship began.

We went on a real date after that first evening together. I was still very hesitant about letting it become serious. However, as he continued to sweep me off my feet, that strict mental checklist of mine became more flexible and our relationship quickly turned into something significant. After just a few dates, we both knew it felt right. He would even tease me about wanting to marry me already. It was so unexpected, especially after dating a couple of other guys who I just couldn't seem to commit to. After just six months of dating, we were ready to move in together.

Here I was, at twenty-seven years old and still hanging on to my virginity. Even though this was by choice, I didn't know anyone else my age who could say the same. This made me feel both proud and excluded at the same time. During my very Christian upbringing, I was taught to follow the bible, which states that sex without marriage is a sin. It didn't help that my mother was a nurse who was very protective, and understandably so. When I was a teenager, she frequently reminded me of the risks that came with being sexually active at a young age. This worry was another reason why I had managed to hold off for as long as I did.

I was always certain that I wanted my first time to be with someone I loved and who loved me in return. I never wanted to be some guy's one-night stand or meaningless hook-up. I felt very strongly about that. However, now that I was in a very committed relationship, and even saw myself potentially marrying this man one day, I felt like it didn't make sense for me to wait any longer. Most women from previous generations were getting married and having kids before the age of twenty. I was twenty-seven years old, and I was with the man I loved.

I will always be proud of myself for maintaining my virginity for as long as I did. It was not easy, especially during my college years when there were so many opportunities to be with different guys. There was a lot of freedom in college, so of course I had fun and enjoyed my share of occasional sleepovers. It was exciting to stay the night with a cute guy I had just met. But most college guys did not want to be in relationships which was understandable. They just wanted to get drunk and have sex with the next hot girl they met at a party. I was in a sorority and liked to go to parties, and I enjoyed being single. However, I never felt the need to sleep around because I knew it wouldn't lead to love and a relationship. As tempted as I was at times, I managed to hold out and preserve my virginity, and I am proud of that.

I had faith that God would forgive me for not waiting until I was married to have sex. He clearly knows that we are all sinners, and he knows that I resisted for as long as I could, longer than most. I waited for the right person, the man I would eventually marry. Therefore, deep down I felt like it was okay to cut myself some slack and that I was deserving of this. Afterall, nobody is perfect, so why did I feel the need to hold myself to that standard?

CHAPTER EIGHT

Ever After

IN OCTOBER 2014, after nearly four years of being together, I got to marry my "Prince Charming." It felt like a fairy-tale wedding. The ceremony was held on the beach just before sunset, with close friends and family, just like I had always imagined. I will never forget the way he looked at me when he first saw me walking down the aisle. There were tears rolling down his cheeks. It was difficult for me to comprehend that this man loved all of me, which included my imperfections and weaknesses. There is no better feeling than the one you get when you have found someone who knows everything there is to know about you, and is still in love with you and wants to be with only you.

Our first year of marriage was not an easy one, as it came with some significant tribulations. The "honeymoon phase" of our relationship had already passed. It wasn't like the old days when our grandparents fell in love and got married right out of high school, and then moved in together, immediately starting a family in their early twenties. We had been dating for three and a half years and already living together for most of that time. Not much really changed once we tied the knot, other than we were officially husband and wife.

Unfortunately, life is not like the fairy tales we see on television or read about in books. Relationships are hard and require a lot of nurturing and compromise. Several months on from our wedding, we came to the decision that a temporary, informal separation was necessary to overcome our struggles and work towards making our marriage a healthy and long-lasting one. This was by far the most painful and emotional experience I had endured. It almost didn't seem real. I felt so alone during this time, even though I knew deep down that I wasn't. I just never saw my life going this way. But life is unpredictable and, thankfully, it didn't last forever. With the help of God, our faith, and, of course, weekly marriage counseling, we were able to find our way back to each other and start rebuilding our life together.

If I learned anything from this time in my life it is that God knows what's best, and he has a plan in store for you even if you can't understand what that may be at the time. Things don't always go the way we want them to. Life is uncertain and full of trials and tribulations. Marriage is not easy, and sometimes there will be roadblocks and hurdles. However, there is always light at the end of the tunnel, and I am so glad that we didn't give up. It was during this time of healing and repairing our relationship that an unexpected blessing came our way.

CHAPTER NINE

My Miracle

I HAVE KNOWN since I was a young girl that I wanted to have kids one day. This was always a significant part of my long-term plan. I hoped to eventually start "trying" for pregnancy once we felt the timing was right. As far as I knew, I was back to optimal reproductive health so I was hopeful that there would not be any issues. Of course, I had no way of knowing for sure, especially given my history. There are lots of couples who have a difficult time conceiving naturally, and some cannot have kids of their own.

We had just gotten back to a good place in our marriage, and back to our normal routine, when I started to notice a change in my body. I didn't know much about pregnancy symptoms, but I knew enough to suspect something when my breasts were suddenly feeling very sore. The fact that I was a few days late in my menstrual cycle raised my suspicion further. I was feeling very scared during this time, but not because I did not want to be pregnant. I just didn't feel ready. I have always been a planner, especially when it comes to significant or life-changing events. We were still healing from our marital challenges, and we were not thinking about starting a family at that moment.

Deep down I already knew the answer to the question that was lingering in my mind. However, I needed proof, and it was important that I did this while I was home alone. So, I drove to the nearest pharmacy and bought a pregnancy test. I still remember the moment I got the result as if it was yesterday. I was finishing my glass of wine, knowing it could possibly be my last for a long time. When I first saw the positive result appear on the test, I was in utter disbelief. Even though it was very evident that it was accurate, due to my symptoms, I couldn't help but wonder if this could be a false test result. But the question I should have been focusing on was did I really want to be pregnant? I had dreamed of becoming a mother since I was little girl. And just a few years prior I had been told that I may not be able to conceive.

On May 7, 2016, just one day before Mother's Day, I gave birth to a beautiful baby girl. She came about four weeks early via an emergency C-section (so much for being a planner). At just five pounds, she was a perfect little angel and my tiny miracle from God. It was an emotional day for me, and obviously physically exhausting, but it will always be the greatest day of my life. My dream of motherhood came true, and I had always envisioned having a baby girl. I already knew what her name would be, and I had known it since I was young.

Becoming a mother for the first time is both exciting and frightening at the same time. Your heart is no longer your own, and you are now responsible for another human's life. I don't believe you can truly understand the meaning and depth of love until you become a parent. It is the most rewarding and natural aspect of life.

CHAPTER TEN

Beautiful Soul

THERE IS NOTHING that can completely prepare you for raising a child these days, especially a daughter. It is very difficult to be a teenage girl and young woman in today's world. Heck, it's even hard to be an "aging" woman these days. There is so much societal pressure when it comes to physical appearance and body image. We live in a world always striving for this mystical idea of "perfection." We see this desire for perfection in everything from our life goals to daily beauty standards, which have become more impossible than ever. So many people are physically changing themselves because they long for this unachievable concept. I am even slightly guilty of this myself.

One day I went to see a plastic surgeon for a consultation to correct my deviated septum. I was so insecure about my nostrils not being perfectly symmetrical. However, he made me realize that it was not necessary. Instead, he offered to change the shape of my nose, which I also was not confident about. As tempted as I was, I knew that I did not want to change a feature that was now a reflection of my beautiful daughter, who inherited this same nose.

The problem is, there is no such thing as being perfect. Our society is striving for an unattainable standard. And to make matters worse, the plastic surgery and cosmetics industry is booming now, and the trend is at an all-time high. There is easy access to Botox, fillers, plastic surgeries of all kinds, and other procedures to change the way we look in a vain attempt to be flawless and ageless. It has even become more affordable, so it is no longer limited to just the wealthy and upper classes, or the "rich and famous." Our culture is dominated by social media, making it so easy to be influenced by others and feel the need to compare yourself and your life to the lives of complete strangers. This can easily become addictive and affect people both mentally and physically in a very unhealthy and negative way. Rather than getting an education and working towards a career, many teens and young adults are now trying to become famous and make a career out of being an "influencer."

Excessive use of social media can be detrimental for any individual, whether male or female, child or adult. It requires self-discipline to limit its use and to remain humble and focused on one's own life and purpose. We all serve a unique, God-given purpose on this earth, and I believe that it has nothing to do with how many followers one has on Instagram, or how young and flawless one may look.

I never want my daughter to go through the same struggles that I went through as a young woman, but I know that this will be difficult to prevent. I want her to understand that imperfection is beautiful and it's what makes each of us special and unique. I want my daughter to love her body and not feel the need to compare herself to others. Again, I know this is easier said than done, because we all tend to want what we don't have, but it is never too early to try and instill this in her. There is so much more to beauty than what is on the outside. For example, having a big, caring, and sensitive heart is a rare yet significant trait. I feel strongly that being a kind person is one of the most attractive qualities someone can have. Life is too short to be so focused on physical appearance.

I was very shy and quiet growing up. I was misjudged, and even bullied for it, in middle school. I was extremely sensitive and cared so deeply about what others thought of me, even though they didn't really know me. I just wanted to be liked by everyone. Despite how hurtful that time was for me, I don't regret it because it helped shape me into the adult that I am today. I realize now that those are the qualities that many people don't have. I am the kind of girl who compliments a stranger or smiles at someone who looks unhappy. I have compassion and kindness, and I truly love that about myself. I didn't understand how important and special that is until I reached my thirties. Grade school has such little significance in the long run.

It makes me sad when I think about how many girls (and perhaps even boys) all over the world battle with some type of body dysmorphia and/or eating disorder, just as I did. We end up punishing our physical bodies due to negative and unrealistic thoughts. One of the things I learned in counseling that truly helped me, as I was battling my own disorder, was to keep a favorite picture of myself, as a little girl, close by. As I felt myself struggling, I would reach for that picture to remind myself of this person, this inner little girl, whom I loved and adored. When I saw myself as that innocent and adorable little girl and realized that she was the same person who I was harming, it made me want to do better. I was treating my body like the enemy, but deep down I cared about myself and did not want to cause harm.

Coming to terms with my flaws, and taking ownership of who I am, did not happen overnight. In fact, it took many years and lots of personal experiences along the way. And, let's face it, I still have my struggles on occasion. After all, I am only human. The body image insecurities don't go away completely. You just learn how to live them in a healthy way.

Learning to become more accepting of myself and my imperfections required a lot of maturity, dedication, and self-care. I also had to learn to recognize, and be okay with, the fact that in this world there will always be another individual who is taller, skinnier, smarter, etc. We must learn to be thankful for the qualities we do have and use those qualities to our advantage. It is not always easy to do, because as humans we naturally tend to fall into the trap of wanting what others have and comparing ourselves to others. We live in such a competitive and materialistic society. However, at the end of the day, we are all mortal and each of us will one day leave this physical life behind, and those things will no longer matter.

It was a long road to becoming someone who, today, I truly admire, love, and respect. With that said, I will never be complacent. I will continue to aspire to be better and do more to make a difference in the lives of others. The way I see it is we will all be somewhat forgotten one day and our physical appearance is only temporary. Having a kind, loving soul and doing good deeds for others can make an impact that will last for eternity. The more people we can serve and love while living on this earth, the more we will be remembered, rewarded, and celebrated in both the physical and the spiritual world.

I will never be a celebrity. I am an average woman who has experienced and grown a lot over the years, and I am one who has come to accept and love her true self. Exercising regularly and eating healthily are still a significant part of my life, but I also let loose and enjoy those occasional pizza and ice cream nights. I have discovered my unique, God-given gifts and how I can use them to help others in a healthcare career that I enjoy. And there is nothing more rewarding than the blessing of motherhood, and being a mother to my daughter brings more purpose and happiness to my life than I could have ever imagined. Until now, I never knew that I would be able to have so much love for a mini version of myself.

There is no such thing as a perfect human being, just like we don't live in a fairy-tale world. Life is meant to be messy, and humans are meant to have flaws. But, if a person could in fact be "perfect," it would be by striving to be the best possible version of their authentic, flawed self. It means embracing everything that makes one beautiful, powerful, and unique. By accepting and owning our imperfections and weaknesses, and making the most of who we genuinely and uniquely are, we can define what is truly human perfection. In other words, less than perfect is truly perfect.

About the Author

LENSEY ACKERMAN is a wife and mother to a young daughter. She is a former Division I college athlete and received a scholarship to play tennis for the University of New Hampshire. She obtained a Bachelor's Degree in Business Administration with a focus in Marketing. As a Director of Marketing in the Assisted Living/ Senior Healthcare industry in South Florida for over 9 years, Lensey is passionate about helping others. She also shares her love for, and knowledge of, health and fitness as a Certified Health Coach.